MORNING PREGNANCY WORKOUT FOR BEGINNERS

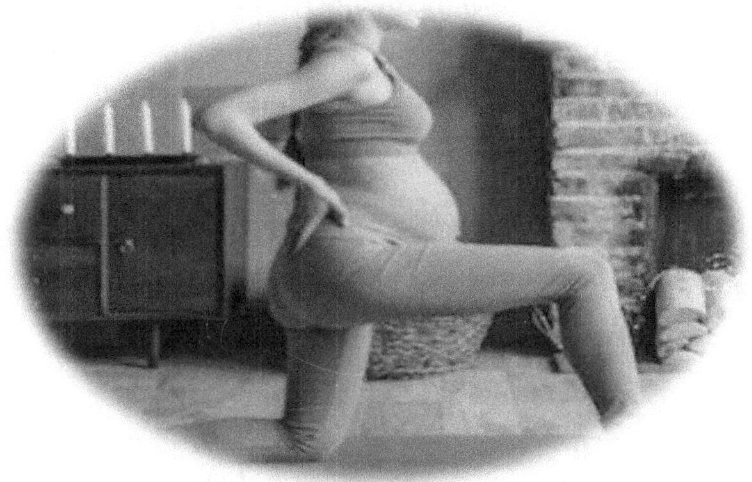

40 Easy and safe morning exercise for healthy pregnant moms to do at home for your baby's development during pregnancy with step-by-step illustrated full body guide to stay fit and happy throughout pregnancy

CARLY EVELYN

SCAN TO GET MORE BOOKS BY THIS AUTHOR

IF YOU ARE STUCK, WHILE PRACTICING THE EXERCISE IN THIS GUIDE, YOU CAN REACH THE AUTHOR AT TRAINERCCARLY@GMAIL.COM FOR GUIDANCE

TABLE OF CONTENT

4)20 MOTIVATIONAL QUOTES FOR MORNING PREGNANCY WORKOUT FOR WOMEN.

5)CONCLUSION

6)PREGNANCY WORKOUT PROGRESS TRACKER IN THE PAPERBACK VERSION

INTRODUCTION

As the first rays of dawn spilled across the horizon, illuminating the quiet town with a soft, golden glow, Emily awoke with a sense of anticipation that tingled through her veins. Today was the day she would embark on a journey that would not only sculpt her body but also cradle the secret growing within her – a morning pregnancy workout plan designed exclusively for women.

With a determined glint in her eyes, Emily slipped into her workout attire, the gentle stretch of the fabric a reminder of the beautiful changes her body was undergoing. The customized routine, a delicate blend of prenatal yoga, low-impact aerobics, and strength training, promised to keep her energized and healthy throughout her pregnancy.

The soft melodies of a specially curated playlist echoed in the room as Emily began her morning ritual. Each movement was a dance, a celebration of the life burgeoning within her. The prenatal yoga poses, gracefully guided by the soothing voice of an instructor through an online video, allowed her to connect with her body and the tiny miracle it harbored.

The low-impact aerobics segment brought a playful rhythm to her routine, with gentle kicks and sways that embraced the essence of pregnancy. Emily felt a surge of endorphins coursing through her, creating a blissful symbiosis between her well-being and the life taking shape within.

As the workout seamlessly transitioned into strength training, Emily marveled at her newfound resilience. The weights, though lighter than her pre-pregnancy sessions, felt substantial, empowering her with a sense of strength that transcended the physical. The instructor's encouraging words resonated through the room, echoing the camaraderie of a womanhood united by the miracle of life.

Completing the morning routine left Emily invigorated, radiating a glow that surpassed the effects of any beauty regimen. She felt connected to her baby in a profound way, as if they had shared an intimate dance, choreographed by the rhythmic beats of the morning workout plan.

In the weeks that followed, Emily's dedication to the pregnancy workout plan became a ritual, a sacred space where she nurtured both her body and the new life burgeoning within. With each passing day, her strength and confidence grew, a testament to the power of embracing the journey of motherhood with mindful exercise.

As Emily continued to weave this captivating dance between her changing body and the curated workout routine, she discovered a profound truth – that in the gentle ebb and flow of each movement, she was not just sculpting her physique but creating a symphony of well-being for herself and the tiny soul nestled within her womb.

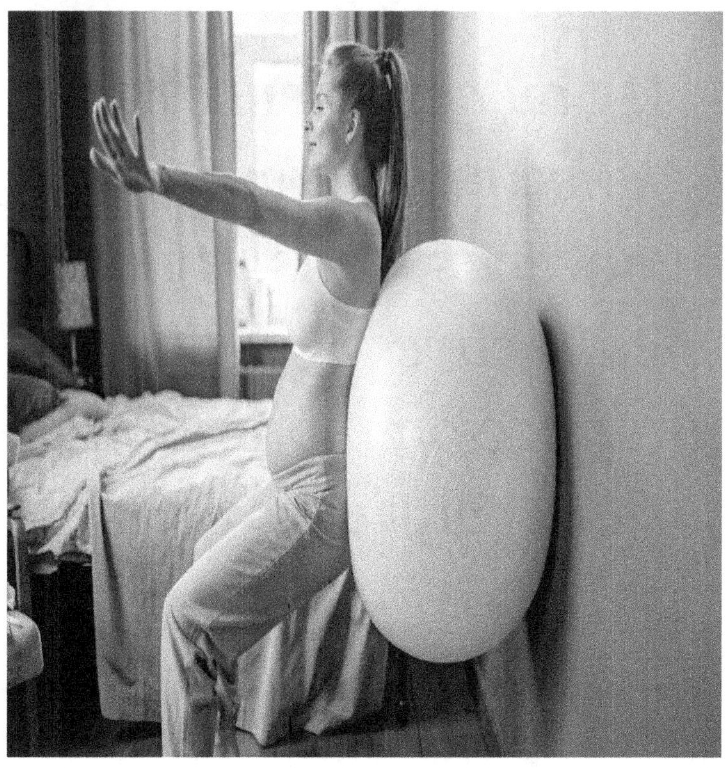

<u>NOTE!!!</u>
Always prioritize safety, comfort, and enjoyment in your pregnancy workouts.

If you experience any discomfort or have concerns, consult your healthcare provider for guidance on modifications or alternative exercises.

STEP BY STEP GUIDE WITH PICTURE ILLUSTRATION

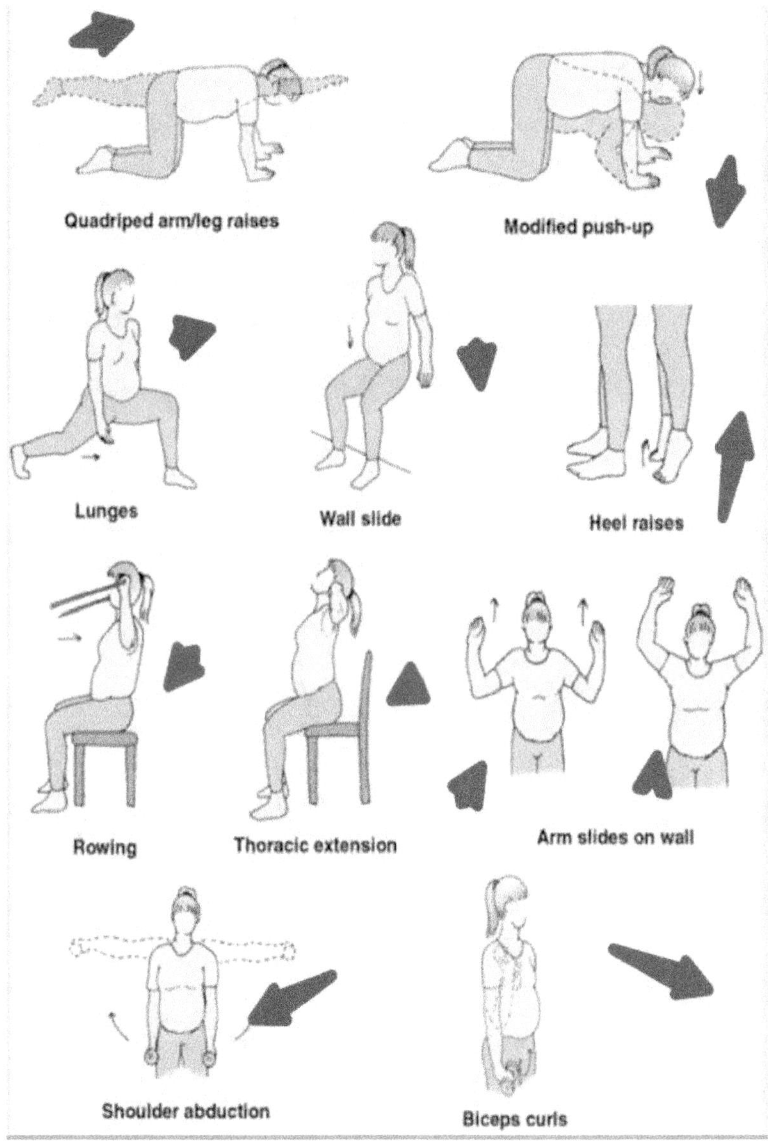

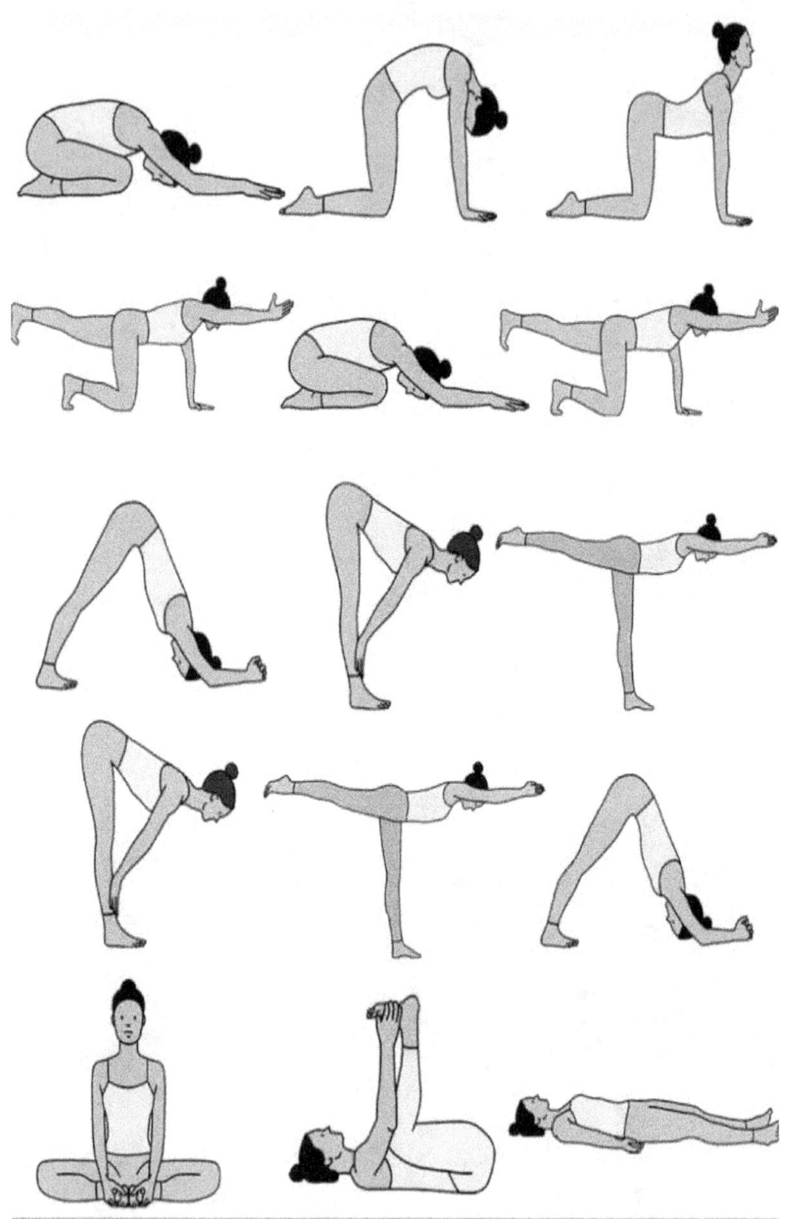

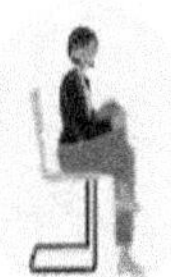

1.Sitting knee lifting with chairs

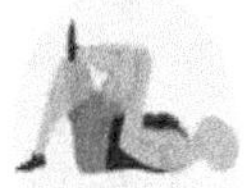

2.Lying side crunches

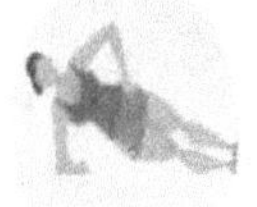

3. Side plank

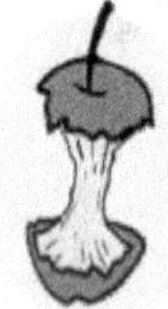

4.Core breath

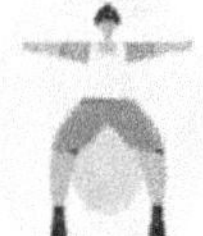

5. Seated stability with ball

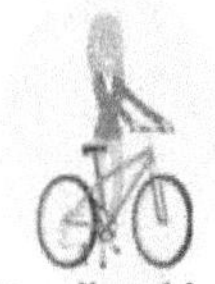

6. Standing bicycle

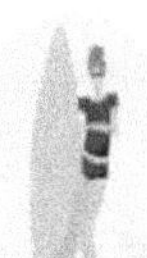

7. Kegels

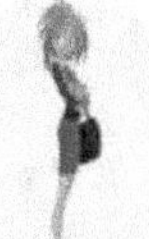

8. Standing crunch

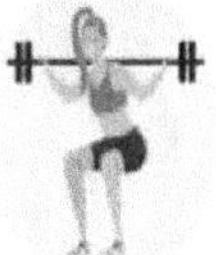

9. Squat

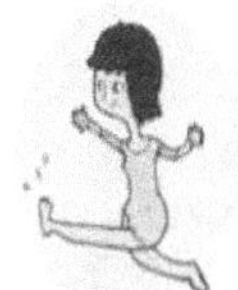

10. Scissor kicks

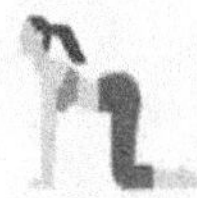

11. Cat cow pose

12. Bird dog

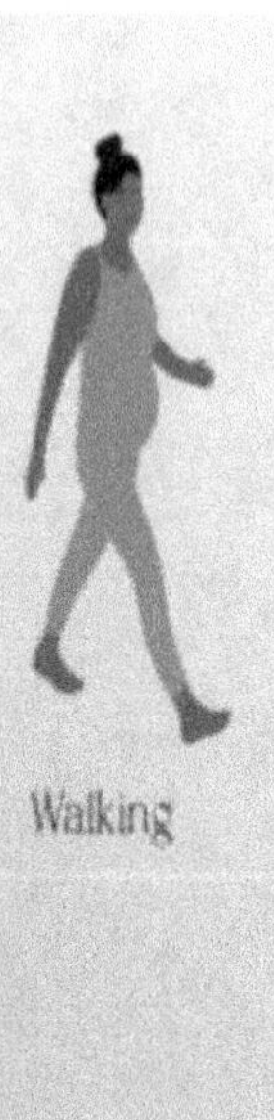

Walking

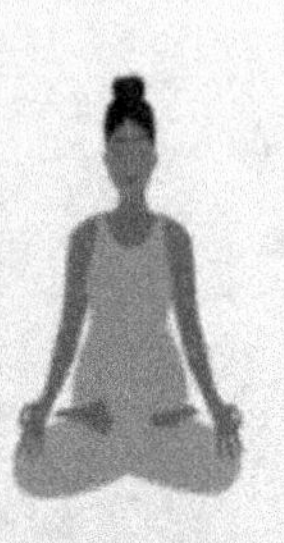

Grounding
Yourself

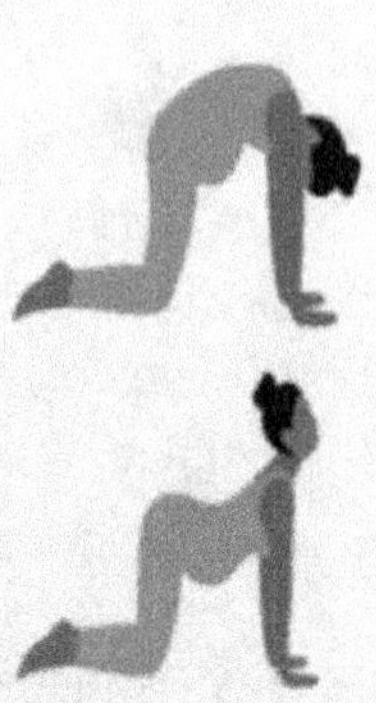

Cat & Cow

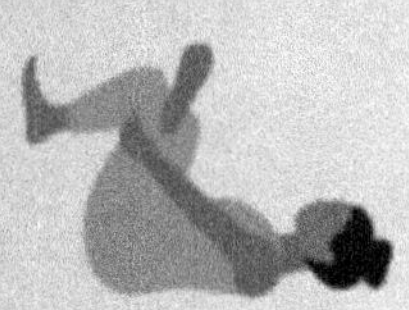

Hip Stretch

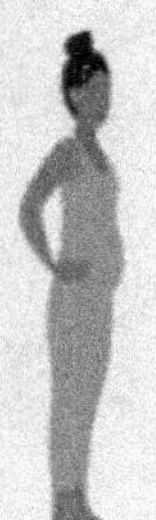

Lunges

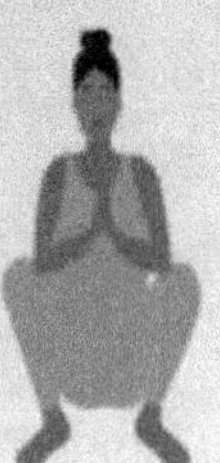

Squats

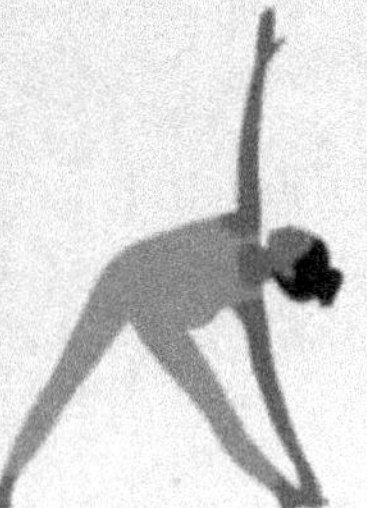

Windmill

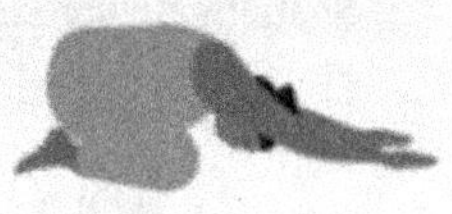

Child's Pose

However, it's crucial to consult with a healthcare professional before initiating any exercise regimen during pregnancy. Individual fitness levels and health conditions may vary, so it's essential to be attentive to your body and adapt exercises as necessary. Below is a varied list of exercises:

1. Pelvic Tilts:
  - **Instructions:**
   - Lie on your back with knees bent.
   - Tighten your abdominal muscles and tilt your pelvis upward, pressing your lower back into the floor.
   - Hold for a few seconds and release.

2. Seated Leg Lifts:
  - **Instructions:**
   - Sit on a chair with your back straight.
   - Lift one leg at a time, extending it straight in front of you.
   - Lower the leg and repeat on the other side.

3. Wall Sit:
  - **Instructions:**
   - Stand with your back against a wall and lower into a seated position.

- Hold for 10-30 seconds, focusing on engaging your thigh muscles.

4. Side-Lying Leg Lifts:
  - **Instructions:**
    - Lie on your side with legs stacked.
    - Lift the top leg while keeping your hips stable.
    - Lower the leg and repeat on the other side.

5. Modified Push-Ups:
  - **Instructions:**
    - Perform push-ups against a wall or on an elevated surface to avoid lying on your stomach.

6. Cat-Cow Stretch:
  - **Instructions:**
    - Get on your hands and knees.
    - Arch your back (cat) and then round it (cow) in a flowing motion.

7. Squats:
  - **Instructions:**
    - Stand with feet shoulder-width apart.
    - Lower your body by bending your knees and hips.
    - Rise back to the starting position.

8. Kegel Exercises:
  - **Instructions:**
    - Contract and relax the pelvic floor muscles.

- Hold each contraction for a few seconds.

9. Arm Circles:
  - **Instructions:**
  - Stand with arms extended.
  - Make small circles with your arms, then reverse the direction.

10. Swimming:
  - **Instructions:**
  - Swim or engage in gentle water aerobics for a low-impact cardiovascular workout.

11. Butterfly Stretch:
  - **Instructions:**
  - Sit with the soles of your feet together and gently press your knees toward the floor.

12. Prenatal Yoga:
  - **Instructions:**
  - Participate in a prenatal yoga class featuring poses suitable for pregnancy.

13. Marching in Place:
  - **Instructions:**
  - Lift your knees alternately while standing in place.

14. Triceps Dips:
   - **Instructions:**
   - Sit on a sturdy chair and place your hands on the edge.
   - Lower your body by bending your elbows and then raise back up.

15. Standing Leg Curl:
   - **Instructions:**
   - Hold onto a chair for support.
   - Lift one foot towards your buttocks, then lower and switch legs.

16. Plie Squats:
   - **Instructions:**
   - Stand with toes turned out.
   - Lower your body into a squat, engaging your inner thighs.

17. Wall Push-Ups:
   - **Instructions:**
   - Stand facing a wall and perform push-ups with your hands on the wall.

18. Bicep Curls:
   - **Instructions:**
   - Use light weights and perform bicep curls while maintaining good posture.

19. Side Plank:
   - Instructions:
   - Lie on your side and lift your body into a side plank position.

20. Modified Jumping Jacks:
   - Instructions:
   - Perform low-impact jumping jacks with a gentle step to the side.

21. Stationary Lunges:
   - Instructions:
   - Take a step forward with one foot and lower your body until both knees are bent.
   - Return to the starting position and switch legs.

22. Bird-Dog Exercise:
   - Instructions:
   - Get on your hands and knees.
   - Extend one arm and the opposite leg, then switch sides.

23. Standing Side Leg Lifts:
   - Instructions:
   - Hold onto a sturdy surface for balance.
   - Lift one leg to the side, then lower and switch.

24. Prenatal Pilates:
   - Instructions:

- Engage in a prenatal Pilates class for a comprehensive full-body workout.

25. Wall Squats:
   - **Instructions:**
   - Stand with your back against a wall and lower into a seated position, holding for 10-30 seconds.

26. Seated Row with Resistance Band:
   - **Instructions:**
   - Sit with legs extended and loop a resistance band around your feet.
   - Pull the band towards you, engaging your back muscles.

27. Prenatal Dance:
   - **Instructions:**
   - Join a prenatal dance class for an enjoyable and rhythmic workout.

28. Standing Calf Raises:
   - **Instructions:**
   - Stand with feet hip-width apart and rise onto your toes, then lower.

29. Leg Press on Stability Ball:
   - **Instructions:**
   - Sit on a stability ball against a wall and press your feet forward.

30. Modified Bicycle Crunches:
   - **Instructions:**
   - Lie on your back with knees bent and perform gentle bicycle crunches.

31. Water Aerobics:
   - **Instructions:**
   - Participate in water aerobics for a buoyant and low-impact workout.

32. Seated Ball Circles:
   - **Instructions:**
   - Sit on a stability ball and make circular motions with your hips.

33. Wall Plank:
   - **Instructions:**
   - Stand facing a wall and lean forward, placing your hands on the wall in a plank position.

34. Inner Thigh Lifts:
   - **Instructions:**
   - Lie on your side and lift the top leg, targeting the inner thigh muscles.

35. Prenatal Cardio Workout:
   - **Instructions:**

- Engage in a prenatal cardio workout routine, such as brisk walking or stationary cycling.

36. Arm Pulses:
  - **Instructions:**
  - Hold light weights and pulse your arms up and down in a controlled manner.

37. Diaphragmatic Breathing:
  - **Instructions:**
  - Practice deep diaphragmatic breathing to enhance relaxation and oxygenation.

38. Prenatal Fitness Ball Exercises:
  - **Instructions:**
  - Utilize a fitness ball for various exercises, such as gentle bouncing and pelvic tilts.

39. Wall Lunges:
  - Instructions:
  - Stand with your back against a wall and perform lunges with proper form.

40. Water Kicks:
  - **Instructions:**
  - Stand in a pool and perform kicking motions for a low-impact leg workout.

1. "Embrace the dawn as you stretch, as each movement in the morning light sculpts not only your physique but also weaves a beautiful tale of strength and the journey into motherhood."

2. "Emerge into the day with radiance; let your morning workout become a joyous celebration of the extraordinary strength dwelling within you, nurturing both your body and the precious life you carry."

3. "With every sunrise, wield the power to shape not only your day but also the bright destiny of the life blooming within you. Let your morning workouts resonate as daily affirmations of your incredible capabilities."

4. "Beyond mere exercises, morning workouts are subtle whispers of empowerment, a profound connection between you and the little one flourishing beneath your heart."

5. "In the serene hush of the morning, discover your inner strength. Each gentle

movement becomes a testament to the unwavering spirit crafting a miracle within."

6. "As the sun caresses the sky, let your workout unfold as a heartfelt letter to your evolving body—a daily dedication to your well-being and the precious life nestled within."

7. "Stir the warrior within – your morning workout transcends routine; it is a proclamation of strength, resilience, and the exquisite beauty inherent in new beginnings."

8. "May the sunrise infuse you with the vigor to carve a masterpiece – not just of your body but of your journey and the miraculous tapestry of life steadily unfolding."

9. "Every stretch, lift, and breath during morning workouts orchestrates a symphony of determination and love, crafting a masterpiece on the canvas of motherhood."

10. "Embrace the potency of the morning, allowing it to fuel your workout. Your body is a canvas, and each movement paints strokes of strength and grace."

11. "Beyond fitness, morning workouts are an avenue to forge a deep connection with the life growing within you. Each graceful move is a dance, a manifestation of love."

12. "In the tranquil dawn, discover your fortitude; embrace your power. Your morning workout is a ritual of self-love, a pledge to the little one blossoming within."

13. "With each sunrise, seize the opportunity to sculpt more than your physique. You're crafting a masterpiece of strength, resilience, and boundless love."

14. "Allow the morning to be your canvas, your workout the brushstroke. Together, they compose a portrait of endurance, courage, and the miracle of creation."

15. "As the sun paints the canvas of the sky, let your morning workout be a brush dipped in determination, sketching the contours of powerful, nurturing motherhood."

16. "Consider the morning your blank canvas; your workout, the artistry of a resilient mother-to-be, shaping a masterpiece with every intentional movement."

17. "In the quietude of the morning, listen to the whispers of your inner strength. Your workout echoes, resonating with the heartbeat of the life burgeoning within."

18. "As the sun extends its rays, allow your morning workout to stretch the boundaries of what you perceive as possible. You possess a strength greater than you realize."

19. "Awaken with purpose, move with intention. Your morning workout is the roadmap to a day filled with strength, energy, and the joy of impending motherhood."

20. "With each morning workout, you aren't merely lifting weights; you're elevating the spirit of resilience and nurturing that will define your journey into motherhood."

21. "The dawn promises a new day; your workout is the vow to embrace it with strength, grace, and the unwavering love of a mother."

22. "In the stillness of the morning, uncover the power within. Your workout is an anthem

of strength echoing through the chambers of your evolving self."

23. "Rise before the sun and let your morning workout be an anthem of commitment – to yourself, your well-being, and the life entrusted to your care."

24. "With the sunrise, renew your commitment to strength, health, and the miraculous journey of pregnancy. Your morning workout is a daily pledge to yourself and your baby."

25. "As the morning light unfolds, so does your potential for strength and endurance. Let each workout be a testament to the incredible power residing within you."

26. "Morning workouts transcend mere perspiration; they're about shattering barriers, pushing limits, and embracing the transformative journey of pregnancy."

27. "With each stretch, you reach beyond physical boundaries—delving into realms of boundless strength, resilience, and the enchantment of motherhood."

28. "In the quietude before the world awakens, let your morning workout be a silent proclamation that today, you are unstoppable, and so is the life within."

29. "With the sun's ascent, you too rise. With your morning workout, you soar. You epitomize the incredible power of a woman embracing the precious gift of motherhood."

30. "Every sunrise gifts a fresh opportunity to sculpt not only your body but also the narrative of a resolute, powerful, and loving mother. Your morning workout is the inaugural brushstroke."

CONCLUSION

In conclusion, this morning pregnancy workout plan for women isn't just a guide to physical fitness; it's an ode to the remarkable journey of motherhood. As you embark on each exercise, remember that you are not merely sculpting your body but also nurturing the beautiful life growing within. The sunrise becomes your accomplice, the morning workout your ritual, and together they form a harmonious symphony of strength, resilience, and boundless love. Embrace the transformative power of these workouts, celebrate the unique connection between you and your growing miracle, and relish the journey into motherhood with every intentional stretch, lift, and breath. May this book be your companion, guiding you with inspiration, support, and the unwavering belief in the extraordinary strength that resides within you. Here's to mornings filled with purpose, vitality, and the radiant anticipation of the beautiful chapter you're crafting—one workout at a time.

PREGNANCY WORKOUT PROGRESS TRACKER IN THE PAPERBACK VERSION

9 798887 368303